Fibromyalgia, Chronic Fatigue and Chronic Illness

Navigating through the confusion and deception, isolating the truly *effective*, science-based treatments to get the <u>real</u> solutions to recover your health and *take back your life!*

By Debbie Baumgarten

Dedication

This book has been a labor of love for many years. It first started as a simple website with information to help others who were suffering as I was. I later decided it really needed to be a manual for those with FMS, CFS and other similar Chronic Illnesses. I know your pain. I know how hard it is. This book is dedicated to you, those who are suffering. From the bottom of my heart, I only hope it can help to ease your pain and misery and improve your quality of life.

Table of Contents

IMPORTANT DISCLAIMER: None of the health topics presented in this book or at **www.fibromyalgiafree.org** have been evaluated or approved by the FDA. They should not replace personal judgment or medical treatment when indicated, nor are they intended to diagnose, treat, cure, or prevent any disease. Always talk to your doctor or naturopathic physician about the use of any of the recommendations for diet, supplements, drugs or exercise or any other complementary modalities.

Introduction

I am not a doctor or a specialist. I am simply someone who has suffered from Fibromyalgia and Chronic Fatigue Syndromes for over 15 years. I also had all of the symptoms of Lupus and Lyme disease, including even the tick-bite and large rash when I was younger and the butterfly face rash that often accompanies Lupus. So for all I know, I may have had any one or all of these chronic illnesses. I was diagnosed with Fibromyalgia, Chronic Fatigue and Myofascial Pain Syndromes at the Mayo Clinic in 2000.

What was the "treatment" for this that one of the top Rheumatologists at the Mayo Clinic recommended? That I take Celebrex. It was a good thing that I didn't follow her advice because Celebrex was later the subject of a class action suit due to serious side effects including causing serious heart problems.

I have tried desperately to find solutions and treatments *that actually work*. I say desperately as it's fifty times harder when you are suffering from debilitating pain and fatigue as well as a host of other symptoms *while* trying to find the answers. And I say "that actually work" because there is a lot of false and misleading information and things that are a waste of time, money and resources that could be put to much better use than lining someone else's pocket.

I have been diligent in my work to recover my former health and vitality. I have done a tremendous amount of research on these subjects, reading tomes of books, blogs and articles.

I have been to numerous clinics from the Mayo Clinic in Florida to the Fibromyalgia Treatment Center in California, The Fibromyalgia and Fatigue Center in Dallas and several others in between.

I have followed numerous protocols and treatments, taken varying types of drugs, tried all manner of supplements, followed a huge array of different diets and exercise programs as well as other therapies and treatments. I was determined to get my life back and I have.

I am also quite convinced that there are many other chronic illnesses that can be effectively treated or at least improved through the application of the information in this book. So if you are suffering from Lyme Disease, Lupus or another similar chronic illness, you too can find relief and possibly even full recovery.

Fibromyalgia and CFS are fairly new. Fifteen years ago there were very few doctors who knew anything about these illnesses and even they knew very little.

Now they have become more known but still no one knows what causes them and, even worse, there are a lot of confusing theories and all kinds of "treatments" including some who are simply trying to profit off the misfortune of others.

This book is simply a synopsis of what I found that, through a lot of trial and error, improved my condition.

My intention is to help those who have been experiencing the many horrible symptoms of these syndromes/chronic illnesses and to hopefully make it possible for you to recover your happy, healthy lives too. If I can save you time and money and connect you to resources that will aid in or help speed your recovery, I will have achieved my goal.

I feel for you. I know what you are going through. And I know how disheartening it can be to be given a wrong diagnosis or wrong treatment. I know what it's like to be told that there is nothing wrong with you or that it's all in your head.

I also know what it's like to be betrayed by false and misleading information and "treatments".

There were times when I hit rock bottom and many times where I felt the despair of having to endure the pain, fatigue and host of other symptoms that are all part of the "Chronic Illness" package. Luckily I have a wonderful husband who has cared for me and helped me through so much. I have also been connected to others on Facebook and support groups that have been so understanding and supportive and have helped tremendously to get me through the rough times. I realized that I had to find the proper balance between cutting myself some slack and kicking myself in the butt to get up and fight for my health. I think it does help to acknowledge that you are in pain, that you are suffering and that life is so much harder in every respect. I think it helps to have others feel for you and empathize.

At the same time, I think there are also times that you have to be just a little bit hard on yourself – hard enough to do the things that are going to make you feel better in the long run.

If you don't, you can go swirling down a dwindling spiral of doing things that appear to comfort you in your agony when in reality they are just making the symptoms worse.

In this book I cover some of the basics about Fibromyalgia and Chronic Fatigue Syndrome, but otherwise I will largely focus on all of the factors that I found to be most important to recovering good health and then maintaining it.

Recovering from these illnesses is not a simple one-shot-in-the-arm treatment. I think we have grown accustomed to going to a doc with our ailment and expecting him to prescribe a pill that fixes it.

Sometimes things are easy like that.

You get some bug, like a bronchial infection and your doctor gives you an antibiotic to take for a week or two, after which you feel better and are able to recover.

If only everything were that easy!

These syndromes are not like that.

I have, over the 15 years that I have known I had Fibromyalgia and CFS, covered a lot of ground on the subject. I have found things that helped, that made a difference and actually improved my condition.

So, I can save you a lot of time by imparting the knowledge I have learned and the many resources I have found. This book is here to provide the information that will allow you to make an informed decision as to whether you might have these illnesses and to give you the right direction as to how to proceed in repairing and freeing yourself from the suffering that accompanies these syndromes.

I sincerely hope that this book will allow many to simply walk their own path out of the emotional darkness that chronic pain and fatigue can bring and help them to return to a healthy and happy life.

A Very Short Overview of These Illnesses

Many of these illnesses have similar symptoms, but they are not exactly the same. Some people, like myself, may be suffering from more than one, as well as some of the co-existing conditions. Sometimes it's hard to tell where one of these illnesses ends and the other begins.

First, let me explain the difference between a syndrome and a disease. A syndrome is a collection of signs and symptoms known to frequently appear together but without a known cause. A disease is characterized usually by an identifiable group of signs and symptoms and a known cause. In short, one has a known cause (disease) and the other doesn't (syndrome).

So realize that while the term "syndrome" sometimes seems to belittle the illness, it's really just a classification based on what the medical establishment *understands* about it. When someone throws out that "it's just a syndrome" argument, they should take a closer look at what they're really saying. It doesn't mean your illness is less real or serious than a disease; it means that it's less understood.

For those of us with these syndromes, it often means many doctors don't know much about them and effective treatments can be hard to find.

Fibromyalgia Syndrome (FMS) in short:

Fibromyalgia is derived from the Greek "algia", meaning pain, "myo", referring to muscle, and the Latin "fibro" meaning the connective tissue of tendons and ligaments.

Fibromyalgia is most definitely very real. Because there is not a specific lab test that shows you have "Fibromyalgia germs", this can tend to be invalidated. However, FMS can be a source of substantial disability.

In 1987 the AMA recognized FMS as a true illness and major cause of disability. The American College of Rheumatology, the American Medical Association, the World Health Organization and the National Institutes of Health have all accepted FMS as a legitimate clinical entity.

In addition to specific tender points, the essential symptom of FMS is pain, although some patients are more troubled by fatigue, soft-tissue swelling, sleep problems and depression.

Here are the main symptoms:

- Widespread pain. Soreness, tenderness, achiness and muscle pain that can last for days, which then finally dissipates and then returns again.

- Sleep problems. Not being able to get to sleep or waking up during the night and not being able to get back to sleep or otherwise restless, disturbed sleep and thus disrupting your ability to get the needed deep sleep that is so vital. This of course contributes to feeling tired and un-refreshed as well as disruption of the body's healing processes and production of vital hormones.

- Fatigue/Exhaustion, which may or may not be connected to the poor sleep. In some cases even despite good sleep one can experience overwhelming tiredness.

- Difficulty with short-term memory or concentration, known as brain fog or fibro-fog.

- Depression, irritability, nervousness and anxiety are often experienced, possibly as a result of the pain and fatigue.

Other common signs and symptoms include:

- Blurred vision or changes in vision.

- Dry and painful eyes.

- Dry membranes in the nose and/or mouth.

- Painful menstrual periods.

- Irritable bowel syndrome (IBS). Constipation, diarrhea, abdominal pain and bloating are often found in people with fibromyalgia.

- Recurrent infections – bladder, urinary tract, eye infections, etc.

- Dry, itchy skin or skin irritations or rash.

A "flare" is a term that refers to the various symptoms of Fibromyalgia flaring up for a matter of hours or more, often for two or three days.

A flare usually follows a period of stress either emotionally or physically or some other factor that can trigger a flare up.

Some examples of triggers could be:

- a night or several nights of very poor sleep
- over-exertion in some physical activity
- working for extended hours
- an increase in caffeine, sugar or alcohol intake
- a long drive or flight
- a long period of time on your feet wearing new or uncomfortable shoes
- a known or unknown infection

These are just some examples of things that can cause a worsening of symptoms.

Chronic Fatigue Syndrome/ME:

Chronic Fatigue Syndrome or "*CFS*" is also at times called Myalgic Encephalopathy or "*ME*", Post-Viral Fatigue Syndrome or "*PVFS*" and Chronic Fatigue Immune Dysfunction Syndrome or "*CFIDS*".

Chronic Fatigue Syndrome/ME is a set of symptoms with severe and almost unrelenting fatigue being most predominant. The fatigue can worsen with physical activity or stress, but it doesn't improve with more rest.

Some of the more common symptoms are: poor sleep, difficulties with short-term memory or concentration, exhaustion after minimal exertion, recurrent infections and bowel disorders. For some, CFS and Fibromyalgia are one in the same.

Chronic Fatigue Syndrome has nine official signs and symptoms:

- Fatigue

- Decrease in memory or concentration

- Sore throat

- Enlarged lymph nodes in neck and/or armpits

- Unexplained muscle pain

- Pain that may move from one joint to another without swelling or redness

- Headache

- Unrefreshing sleep

- Extreme exhaustion lasting more than 24 hours after physical or mental exertion

Lyme Disease

Lyme Disease is transmitted through a tick bite that has one of several bacterial infections and transfers the bacteria through his bite.

Often, but not always, the bite will result in a rash around the bite site.

When this infection is caught early enough it can be treated with antibiotics. If not caught and treated early on, the disease can progress into more serious symptoms.

Lyme disease can cause flu-like symptoms, with muscle and joint pain and swollen lymph glands. It can also result in severe fatigue, headaches, arthritis, other inflammation and sometimes nerve damage.

Lyme disease symptoms can also be improved with the various protocols listed in this book.

Lupus

Lupus is a chronic inflammatory syndrome that occurs when your body's immune system attacks your own tissues and organs. Inflammation caused by lupus can affect your joints, skin, kidneys, blood cells, brain, heart and lungs.Lupus can be difficult to diagnose because the signs and symptoms are often very similar to those of other ailments, such as the ones I've already listed. The most distinctive sign of lupus — a facial rash that resembles the wing of a butterfly across each cheek — occurs in many but not all cases of Lupus.

The underlying cause of Lupus is also unknown.

Symptoms vary from person to person, and may come and go. Almost everyone with Lupus has joint pain and swelling and some develop arthritis. Frequently affected joints are the fingers, hands, wrists, and knees. Other common symptoms include:

- Chest pain when taking a deep breath

- Fatigue

- Fever with no other cause

- General discomfort, uneasiness, or ill feeling (malaise)

- Hair loss

- Mouth sores

- Sensitivity to sunlight

- Skin rash - a "butterfly" rash on the face sometimes occurs

- Swollen lymph nodes

Co-existing conditions:

There are numerous other physical conditions that may accompany FMS, CFS, Lyme disease and Lupus. Some of these are:

A) *Chronic Myofascial Pain Syndrome*: Very often with the above listed illnesses someone can also have Chronic Myofascial Pain (CMP) as a co-existing condition. Myofascial pain is probably the most common cause of musculoskeletal pain in medical practice. Fascia is the thin, translucent film that wraps around muscle tissue, blood vessels, nerves, lymph glands and even your organs. The outer layer of fascia is attached to the underside of your skin. Capillary channels and lymph vessels run through this layer and so do many nerves.

If this layer of fascia is healthy, then your skin can move fluidly over the surface of your muscles.

In FMS and CMP this fascia is often stuck and this is where there is great potential to store excess fluids and metabolites. The deeper layer of this fascia covers your internal organs and surrounds the blood vessels, lymph vessels and nerves. Changes of pressure due to the compression by tightening myofascia can affect the cells that lie within the blood, lymph vessels and nerves. Another form of fascia surrounds and protects the spinal cord and contains the spinal fluid. It is also connected to the membranes that surround your brain and together they hold and protect your craniosacral system. It is the tightening of this fascia that restricts blood flow.

B) *A Compromised Immune System*:
Resulting in unknown infections also often accompanies FMS, CFS, Lyme and Lupus.

These can include bacterial infections, viruses or viral infections, yeast infections and even parasites. Urinary tract/bladder infections, sinusitis, eye infections, numerous viruses, walking pneumonia and many other examples of infections can result from a compromised immune system that often exists with chronic pain and fatigue sufferers.

C) *Irritable Bowel Syndrome*: This is also common. This is where the muscles in the gut contract and relax at the wrong time resulting in gas, bloating, constipation and/or diarrhea.

D) *Restless Leg(s) Syndrome (RLS)*: RLS is a neurological disorder characterized by throbbing, pulling, creeping, or other unpleasant sensations in the legs and an uncontrollable urge to move them. Symptoms occur primarily at night when a person is relaxing or at rest and can get worse during the night.

E) *TMJ*: The temporomandibular joint is a hinge that connects your jaw to the temporal bones of your skull, which are in front of each ear. It lets you move your jaw up and down and side-to-side, so that you can talk, chew, and yawn. Problems with your jaw and the muscles in your face that control it are known as Temporomandibular Disorders (TMD). However you may hear it called TMJ.

After reading all of these over you can see that there are many symptoms that overlap and often it is hard to tell what is causing what or where one disease/syndrome or condition ends and another one begins.

I had the butterfly rash on my face for quite some time but was never diagnosed with Lupus. I have also been bitten by ticks, including one that produced a large rash, but blood tests that were done indicated that I did not have Lyme Disease.

Finally, I realized that it didn't much matter what my exact diagnosis was as there were no definite cures for any of them. What I did know was that I felt horrible and I had to do something.

So I saw lots of docs, got lots of tests and did more and more research and studies to find answers that could bring some relief.

The Horrible Trap

There is a trap that I fell into numerous times and that I see many others afflicted with these illnesses fall prey to because it is so easy to do. This is the vicious cycle where you feel bad, you are in pain, you are tired, you have to go to work or you have children that need to be cared for or some form of responsibilities to take care of. So you do something to give yourself enough pick-me-up to be able to get through the day – coffee, a coke, a souped-up Starbucks latte, some sweets, a Red Bull, some carbs, maybe even a cigarette or some combination of the above. This might buck you up for a bit and help you to get through some short-term period but, in the longer run, you have made matters worse. With all of the extra insulin your body just pumped in response to what you put in it, you will worsen the fatigue and pain and you may get poor sleep to boot.

Now you are even more desperate for some form of pick-me up because now you feel even worse.

Of course you don't feel like exercising, as you just don't have the energy and/or you are in a lot of pain already.

Continuing on in this vein will cause more and more despair and depression, as you feel terrible, you are desperate to get some energy and the quick energy sources are making matters worse and worse. Or, you are so depressed about the situation or the continuous pain that you comfort yourself with things you think will make you feel good – comfort food, alcohol, cigarettes or some form of drugs (OTC or otherwise).

This is what I call a vicious cycle. Things are bad, and the quick and available fixes just make it worse. If you are in such a situation, there IS a way out. It isn't instant.

It takes some time. It isn't horrifically slow either. However it will take some dedication and discipline. The first step is to gain an understanding of what is happening and what you need to do.

As you treat some of the underlying real causes of your condition and start to feel better, you will be able to phase out other drugs that are just masking the symptoms (and making things worse in the longer run) as well as other crutches such as comfort foods, alcohol, nicotine, etc. This should be done as soon as possible, but don't rush it either.

I recommend one at a time. Several times I was zealous enough to try doing it all at once – stop smoking, stop all sugar, simple carbs and all meds. It never worked.

I would lose it within several days. It was too much at once. It's best to pick one, maybe the easiest one, and cut it out or even gradually wean off of it and get to a point where you can stably stay off of it.

I don't recommend trying to do this until you have progressed through a number of the other steps of this program. You should be sleeping well fairly consistently and at least be getting some good nutrition through a healthy diet and supplements. As you start feeling a little better, it is easier to phase these out gradually.

Things like caffeine and sugar consumption can be gradually weaned. Some things are more, such as cigarettes or even alcohol, these probably should be stopped cold as soon as possible.

To quit smoking, there are resources, such as nicotine patches and a book I highly recommend called *The Easy Way to Stop Smoking*", by Allen Carr. Consult your doctor regarding any prescription medications. See my later chapter on this subject.

I just want to make sure you understand that these crutches that you think are comforting you or helping you to endure the pain and misery that you are going through are actually making matters worse. And they will need to be ousted from your life one by one if you truly want to regain your health.

False and Misleading Information and Treatments

It is my opinion that most of the promoted drugs "for Fibromyalgia" only serve to mask the symptoms and do nothing to treat any of the underlying causes. And these drugs have side effects that can just end up complicating the situation further.

Ever notice how a lot of the commercials for these great wonder-drugs on TV spend way more time explaining the horrible side effects of their drug (while playing pleasing music and showing you images of happy people) than they do telling you what the drug is supposed to do – and that's only done to protect themselves from lawsuits as a result of those horrible side effects so they can say "we warned you". Nevertheless, it makes the point that they aren't all they are cracked up to be.

Taking these medications may treat the symptom it is designed for but, at the same time, it may cause another ailment. For example, Prozac, a commonly used medication for treating depression, lists fatigue and insomnia as a common side effect.

Doctors often prescribe painkillers for the pain, anti-depressants for the mood swings or depression, sleeping pills so you can get to sleep at night (and you may even have to take uppers to wake up in the morning). Often these types of medications are necessary to manage symptoms on a short or medium-term basis. Long-term use of such meds can have some serious downsides.

I am not telling you not to follow something your doctor prescribes. Please follow sound medical advice. I am not a doctor. My main concern, that I want you to keep in mind about these drugs, is that this is a degenerative condition.

If this is the only route you chose to take, be prepared to be washing down ever increasing amounts of life-numbing drugs for many years to come.

What's best here is to focus on how to lessen the symptoms by addressing their root causes and thus reduce the dependency or continued need for these drugs. There are a few people around that are trying to make a profit on our misery. Like some of these promoted drugs, various treatments and other supplements for FMS, CFS or other Chronic Illnesses -- many of which I tried – they were a waste of time and money due to lack of results.

Somehow throughout all of this, try to be more skeptical or even cynical of promoted magic pills or treatments, while also somewhat open to new things. Question things before you jump. Research them, read reviews and any info you can find on something before you invest your valuable time and money into it.

A Workable Strategy to Recover your Health

One thing I like to know when I am reading a book on a subject like this is what the overview is as to where this book is going. This helps to tell me if this is something I am interested in or is it just a rehash of information I have read numerous times.

If it looks like it is along the lines of what I have found to be true and yet offers some new information or new angle on things that I may not know about, I am particularly excited and driven to read the book as intensively as possible. So here is a basic overview of where I am going with this book and how I hope to be of help to you. It's basically the strategy that I eventually formulated (after a lot of trial and error) to get well and recover from these illnesses and stay well.

In the chapters to follow, there is detailed information on exactly how to do each of these steps.

However this gives you an idea of where we are going.

- Improve sleep with ways to get a better night's sleep to aid in healing.
- Bump up the nutrition – this book contains a very short synopsis of what I have found to be most important with regards to your diet that will help you feel better.
- Lightening your stress load as much as you possibly can.
- With the help of a competent doctor, isolating any active bacterial, viral or yeast infections or infectious diseases and following an appropriate regimen to either kill these bugs or get them

under control by the body's own defense system.

- Implementing a natural approach to addressing viruses and infections without the use of drugs.
- Further building up and strengthening your immune system so as to keep those at bay.
- Get your hormones properly balanced. Problems such as low thyroid or estrogen dominance can be causing or worsening some of your symptoms.
- As you start feeling better, begin phasing out pain and sleep meds, antidepressants (which should all be done under a doctor's supervision), cut back on sugar and other comfort foods, as well as any other crutches so to speak, such as alcohol, caffeine, nicotine, etc.

- Avoid known triggers that can cause symptom flare-ups
- Start exercising daily, even if it is the lightest possible bit of exercise. Start very light and slow and build up gradually.
- Meanwhile stay on a healthy diet, continue supplements and any needed bio-identical hormone therapy, get good sleep, stay away from high stress situations as much as you can. At this point you are in maintenance mode in a much healthier and more operational state.

You don't have to do this exact sequence but I think this is probably best. For example, you could start exercising right away. Exercise (as long as it is not overdone) helps a lot to decrease pain and increase energy and metabolism.

The only problem is that when I felt so

horrible, I just could not get myself to exercise on a regular basis. Once I was feeling a bit better, then I was able to start light exercises on a daily basis and keep doing it.

That's why I have exercise toward the end of the list, but certainly it wouldn't hurt to do this earlier.

The more of this strategy that you employ, the easier it gets to do more, as each one helps to improve matters. Hopefully with the more detailed information given in the text of this book, I can make it a bit easier for you to take the right steps to get well.

Also, please realize that there may be a lot of ups and downs on this road to recovery. One of my doctors drew me a little diagram to demonstrate what to expect. He drew a wave that went up and down and up and down but with the overall trend leading in an upward direction.

It was good for me to have that picture and know what to expect, as then I didn't have a tendency to throw in the towel when I had bad days or hit a rough patch.

If over time your "downs" aren't as low as they were a month or two ago and your "ups" are higher, then you know you are headed in the right direction.

An Important Step When Embarking on Recovery

Before I go further in this book, there is one thing I would like to ask you to do and that is to keep a really simple daily log or journal.

The reason is that you can gain a wealth of information about yourself and your treatment by doing this one simple step. You will be able to tell what things help your condition and what factors cause adverse reactions. You will be surprised how just trying to do it from memory can result in not getting it quite right and forgetting important details.

I will make this as simple as possible, but you will need to make a conscious effort to do this daily.

What worked best for me was a small notebook next to my bed that I filled out each night.

I made a little list (like the one below) of the important points to make note of and put it on the inside front cover so I could refer to it each time.

Sleep – quality and quantity.

Meds – any changes in medications or supplements.

Diet changes – note any major changes.

Triggers – sugar, alcohol, travel, etc.

Exercise – what kind and how much.

Pain levels –for that day.

Fatigue levels – for that day.

Anything else of note.

You can either keep a simple record in a notepad or you can download and use an application to keep track of these details.

Apps such as *"FibroMapp"* or *"Chronic Pain*

Tracker" can be used if this is easier for you.

It takes 1-2 minutes and is well worth the effort.

Later you can review these and get a lot of good information such as supplements that helped, diets you did better on, triggers you weren't aware of and other valuable tweaks for your program.

Immediate Means of Relief

There are a number of ways that I have successfully relieved pain and other symptoms on a short-term basis and these should certainly be in any fibro-warrior's arsenal. There's nothing very profound or earthshattering in this section and most likely you have already discovered some or all of these, but just in case, I will list what I know.

Hot Bath*:* I love a hot bath when I am achy or just feel bad. It really helps to relieve pain for hours or sometimes can even cool a flare down completely. I always use a very healthy amount of Epsom Salts or other Mineral Salts that have a ton of magnesium. Magnesium is a natural muscle relaxant and I think it is best when absorbed through the skin directly into the blood stream, rather than only through the digestive tract. I also put some lavender essential oil in as well, which smells so good, to make this a feel-good-fest. I also add hot water periodically to keep it at a nice hot temp. Inevitably the pain eases down but sometimes you don't realize how much until after the bath when you are laying in bed and you realize the pain has come down at least several notches.

Hot Shower: A long hot shower can really help. What's good about a shower is that you can let the water run over your head, neck and back. I like to do a little gentle stretching of my neck muscles and sideways stretching of my back while under the hot water. As you get more used to the water temperature you can periodically increase the heat a bit to a really hot but pleasant level.

In both cases, hot bath and shower, I recommend making sure the bathroom is well heated (I use a little space heater) to keep you warm during your soak and so you don't get cold when you get out.

Muscle Creams*:* such as Arnica Cream can also help. There are a ton of brands and options on this. I don't like using creams that are full of chemicals and unnatural things that go right into my bloodstream through my skin. ProSirona, MyoNatural Pain Cream and Rub On Relief are some options you might try.

Heat*:* Heat can often help achy muscles. For inflammation you should use cold, like an ice pack that is covered. For sore or achy muscles, heat works great. There are numerous ways you can get heat into your muscles. Of course a hot bath or shower provides lots of wet heat and I have found wet heat to be very helpful. But sometimes while we are working or doing other things, having some additional heat into those achy muscles can really help. Here are some things you can do:

- Heating pad – which you can put over your back or shoulders. I have an extra long one that works great.

- Thermacare Heat Packs – I love these. They have different shapes and sizes. They are great to put on under your clothes and usually last for 8 hours or longer. I use them on my back and shoulders or a particularly achy joint.
- Infrared Sauna: I bought a great little infrared sauna on Craigslist for a greatly reduced price. The infrared seems to get the heat deeper into my muscles and this really helps. I do some stretching and then spend 20-30 minutes in the sauna and love it.

Rest or Naps: I use to always battle my fatigue and force myself to push through it (which I don't recommend). When it was so bad that I finally relented and took a nap, I would often pass out for a couple of hours. Afterwards I felt less fatigued but felt really out of it and would always have a hard time sleeping that night.

This made me more resistive to napping. However, what I have found that works well is either a) just lying down and resting (watching a show on TV or a video on my computer) or b) taking a short nap for like 15 or 20 minutes where I don't go into a deep sleep. I have my husband wake me or set my phone to buzz after 20 minutes. Either of these has helped to refresh me and ease off the fatigue without adversely affecting my sleep that night.

Therapeutic Massage: I think any kind of massage helps ease some pain by improving blood flow through the muscles. Of everything I have tried, I have gotten the greatest benefit from an actual massage therapist who hones in on trouble spots and really works out the kinks in those more painful or locked up areas. I also like deep tissue massages as long as they don't go too hard. If you prefer something softer and more relaxing, a Swedish massage can be great too.

Trigger point therapy and Myofascial release are two additional methods that you may find helpful or relieving. I think you should try different ones and find what works best for you.

For Christmas my brother bought me a Brookstone massager and this is really easy to use on my neck and back. Since I don't have the funds to get professional massages that often, this little machine has been a godsend.

Chiropractic Adjustments: I have been to a lot of chiropractors and have tried a number of different theories and techniques. I often experienced a lot of pain when being adjusted which I, of course, didn't like. When I tried gentler methods I didn't really experience much relief. For a while I gave up, but later I found a happy place with chiropractic.

I found that if I either got a really good massage before getting an adjustment the chiropractor could adjust me much more gently with very good results. Also if I or the chiropractor massaged the muscles around the spine well this helped too.

For me, I found one out of probably ten different chiropractors that I did well with. Once I found one that worked for me, I have been able to get an adjustment from him when I need it and it really helps to bring down pain.

If you try chiropractic, I recommend being vocal about what you can tolerate and working with him or her to find the right techniques and level of force that works best for you.

Acupuncture: This is something that I am embarrassed to say I have never tried as I just get a bit weirded out about lying there with a bunch of needles stuck in me. Anyway, because I have heard from many others that acupuncture can be very helpful, I thought it really should be included in this section.

OTC Anti-Inflammatory or Sleep Meds: I
used to heavily depend on these to ease pain so
that I could keep working and to get a good
night's sleep. I have popped a lot of Advil and
OTC sleep meds in my day.

Being that they were over-the-counter, I could
get an endless supply of them.

What I hadn't done was read the fine print on
the box, the warnings about long-term use and
the clear instructions that you are only
supposed to take them for a short period of
time. Since then I have read up on the dangers
and bad side effects of long term use of
NSAIDs, Tylenol, etc.

So while they can provide short-term pain
relief, I have stopped using them at all unless I
really have to on a very rare occasion.

Here is an article (one of many if you search on
the Internet) that you should read that gives
some very good information on this.

This article compares taking over-the-counter pain meds to playing Russian roulette after a survey of over 175 million people who take over-the-counter pain relievers found that more than half of them admitted to exceeding the recommended doses and very few of them were aware of the risks, which include stomach bleeding, ulcers and other serious risks.

This article also states,

> *"Although most nonprescription pain relievers are safe for healthy people when used as directed, some of the most commonly used medications, known as NSAIDs or nonsteroidal anti-inflammatory drugs, can cause potentially deadly side effects.*
>
> *NSAIDs include aspirin and drugs containing ibuprofen or naproxen,*

such as Advil and Aleve.

"Researchers say 16,500 people die and 103,000 are hospitalized each year because of NSAID-related problems."

Later in the article it says,

"The risk is considerably higher for older adults, especially for women who frequently take the drugs for persistent pain."

This described me – a woman in my fifties taking these meds pretty much every day for persistent pain.

The point being, these drugs are not intended to treat chronic pain – read the fine print in the warning labels.

So maybe you need to take over-the-counter pain meds for a short time, but it is vital to have a healing protocol in place so that you can phase out taking these as rapidly as possible.

A similar danger is in use of OTC sleep meds, most of which are antihistamines, in that they have been linked to Alzheimer's and dementia. I cover more information on this, as well as alternative aids to help you sleep, later in this book.

Battling Depression

There is a common symptom that goes along with Fibromyalgia/CFS (as well as other chronic illnesses such as Lyme Disease and Lupus) and that is depression. Of course you don't have to be suffering from a chronic illness to get depressed – anyone can experience depression. Sometimes it comes and goes and sometimes it is chronic and unrelenting.

Here are the things that I have found that have helped to pull me out of it when I have fallen into that dark, deep pit.

1. B vitamins help tremendously. You can get B Complex 100 or you can get B vitamins from natural sources such as nutritional yeast, brewers yeast, molasses, turkey, tuna, liver, legumes, whole grains, bananas and chili peppers.

I recommend getting your B vitamins from both types of sources as we are talking fairly high doses. In addition to consuming foods that are rich in B vitamins, I also take three or four B-complex capsules spread out throughout the day. Don't take them on an empty stomach – take with food or yogurt.

2. Get out into the environment – take a walk, sit on your patio, do something to get your attention out of your head and out into the environment. Make a point to look around at the trees, the sky, or the birds. Find some beauty in your environment.

3. Do physical work – yard work, house cleaning, repair something, build something or do other household chores. Again, do something that gets you out of your head and puts your attention out on the environment. Don't over-exert yourself as that could make you feel even worse later, so just do light work.

4. De-clutter something – your office, your papers, your pantry, anything that is cluttered. De-cluttering can be very therapeutic.

5. Do something to help someone. There is no better way to improve your mood than doing something kind or helpful for another.

6. Do something creative – play any form of music, make a flower arrangement, paint, draw, make pottery or anything that you enjoy that involves some sort of creativity.

None of these are easy to do when you are feeling down. However, if you can get yourself to do at least one of these, then maybe you will feel up to doing another one.

Sooner or later, I think you will find some relief.

Improve Your Quality of Sleep

Getting a good night sleep is how your body recovers from stress and activity during the day. It makes a world of difference in your energy level and performance the next day. It's vital to having a strong immune system. Being tired can also encourage unhealthy "solutions" due to sugar cravings, caffeine cravings and other quick-energy desires, just because you are trying to give your body an extra jolt to compensate for being tired.

There are some things that can help your quality of sleep. Melatonin is one. This is a hormone that you can get in most health food stores or areas where vitamins are sold. I use the kind that is time released as I use to have a problem of waking up during the night and not being able to get back to sleep. You need to find the right dose that works best for you. I use 5 mg time released.

My brother takes twice that amount. My husband, when he uses it, takes a much smaller dose.

Sleep schedule: Having a stable sleep schedule helps a lot too. You need to find your sleep schedule sweet spot. I tend to wake up early, so I have found it is best for me to go to sleep around 10 or 10:30 at night. I wake up at 6 or 6:30am with a good night's sleep. If I stay up much later than that I usually find I get a crappy night of sleep. If you want to sleep later in the morning past sunrise, then I recommend black out curtains or shades to keep the room dark. There are also things that can trigger a bad night's sleep. Consuming a lot of MSG (Monosodium glutamate – a flavor enhancer that is sometimes put into food) can be one. Another trigger is alcohol. Caffeine or dark chocolate late in the day or evening, as they are stimulants, can keep you from going to sleep or sleeping restfully.

If none of the above easy remedies help you sleep, then please don't resort to taking over-the-counter sleeping meds. A new study has found a definite link between the use of anticholinergic drugs (including popular non-prescription sleep aids and antihistamines such as diphenhydramine) and an increased risk of developing dementia and Alzheimer's disease. Here's a link to one of many articles on the subject:

http://www.medicalnewstoday.com/articles/288546.php

In this article, it explains that,

> ***"The higher the cumulative amount of drug taken, the higher the risk of developing dementia."***

In other words, a very rare or occasional use is less risky, but long term repeated use can greatly increase the risk of dementia – and that is not something you want to gamble with.

There is another solution that may be applicable to many women with consistent sleep issues. It completely handled my sleep problems (which started just as I was headed toward menopause). Progesterone in capsules or caplets, which must be prescribed by a doctor, that you can take each night at bedtime. You can also use a cream, but I found that taking it orally was much better for sleep.

Of course this would require proper hormone testing and a doctor's prescription, but it is well worth the trouble if you aren't sleeping well and usual supplements don't help.

It's also much better than over-the-counter sleep meds.

The Damaging Effects of Stress

Stress can come from many things. There is physical stress on the body – this can come from an injury or accident, disease, surgery, having to endure severe conditions, extreme weather conditions, extreme physical exertion, physical exertion for too long, sleep deprivation and many other examples of physical stress.

There is also mental stress. When our jobs, livelihood, family or our possessions are in danger or there is a threat of loss we usually experience stress.

There are many different types of stressors. An accident or injury can be an extreme stress on one's body and mind. Other sudden events can be incredibly stressful. The death of a loved one, an unexpected lawsuit, loss of a home or business or job, being told that you or a loved one has a life-threatening disease or situation, a heavy viral or bacterial infection or illness. These and many more examples all cause varying levels of stress.

There is also the type of stress that isn't as severe, but that is long-term. A stressful life or work relationship or circumstances can go on for months or even years, taking its toll and wearing your defenses down.

One doesn't have to be the VP Sales for some huge corporation to be under stress. You might work for a small company and simply have a mean, grumpy boss or, worse, a somewhat sadistic boss or co-worker, and you can be under a lot of stress as a result of repeated antagonism toward you. Maybe your commute to and from work is treacherous or stressful due to traffic or other conditions. Or maybe you have some relationship at home that is stressful.

It could be that home is fine and you love work but you aren't making enough financially to cover your expenses and so you are stressed about your own or your business finances.

These and countless other scenarios can be causing you extra stress.

Stress causes a cascade of reactions and changes in your body including many hormonal changes.

Stress, in some form or another, is usually what activates Fibromyalgia – initially at onset of the disease, as well as full relapses of it and short-term flare-ups.

Also one's reaction to stress varies from person to person. For example, some people don't mind speaking in front of an audience, whereas some people find it incredibly stressful. So your attitude or reaction to potentially stressful situations plays a part in it as well.

It can also be that you aren't fully aware of how much stress you are experiencing. Some people consider it part of life or "normal" to be under stress. But the truth is that it isn't healthy to be under stress for any length of time.

Stress, particularly prolonged stress that goes for weeks, months or even years, can be very taxing on your body and can cause quite some damage.

When you are stressed your adrenal glands are forced to produce more cortisol and adrenaline (the main stress hormones) than usual. These hormones rouse the body for emergency action. Your heart pounds faster, muscles tighten, blood pressure rises, breath quickens, and your senses become sharper. These physical changes increase your strength and stamina, speed your reaction time, and enhance your focus—preparing you to either fight or flee from the danger at hand.

Stress that continues over long periods of time and is left unchecked can contribute to health problems, such as high blood pressure, heart disease, obesity and diabetes. Stress can also trigger or re-trigger FMS or CFS.

Because of the widespread damage stress can cause, it's important to know your own limit.

It is also vital that you work to reduce stress in your life in every way you can. There are several approaches to this that can help.

Part of reducing stress can come from your attitude toward the stressful situations. Talking about it with someone can often help. Meditation and other self-help techniques can also go a long way in reducing stress.

Sometimes it is just a matter of certain people in your environment that cause you stress. This can be a rough relationship with your spouse or another family member, a neighbor, a co-worker or boss, someone from a group that you frequent, etc. If it is a neighbor or co-worker and you can somehow reduce contact with that person, then this might help in relieving that tension.

If it's your boss or spouse or other family member, then talking about the situation with someone else can sometimes help. Talking about it with the person directly, where this is possible, can also often help. You can get professional help to address the matter, or maybe it's time to get a new job or lay down some new ground rules in the house.

Perhaps you can make an appeal to people close to you. Explain that stress is a trigger for your illness and ask for their help to keep relationships calm and do what they can help lower your stress levels. If they understand that there are physical consequences to stressful situations, they may be willing to work with you to help you recover.

Sometimes particular situations can cause stress, such as debt load resulting from not making enough money to adequately cover expenses. This might require confronting the details of the situation and coming up with a real way of handling such as budgeting your expenditures to fit within available funds and then honestly enforcing this budget be followed by all concerned.

In other words, maybe there is a real situation that you are facing that needs confronting and to have real solutions worked out.

Just isolating where your stress is coming from can be very enlightening and relieving. Once you really nail down where your stress is coming from, then it isn't hard to work out immediate, medium and long-range handlings for it.

Exercise that is Extraordinarily Easy and Builds Slowly

My favorite exercise program is the Royal Canadian Air-force Exercise Plan. Actually there are two plans; one for men and one for women.

Written more than 50 years ago, these are simple exercise routines that anyone can do without any additional equipment. These routines are usually done in less than 10 minutes, or 12 minutes max. They start on a very, very low level of exertion and increase in number of repetitions as well as required strength and agility on a very gradual basis, which you increase at your own speed.

You can download the two booklets – one for men (5BX) and one for women (XBX) at my website: **fibromyalgiafree.org/fibromyalgia-and-exercise.**

Read all of the information in the beginning of the booklets so that you understand the theory of these exercises and how the whole plan works.

If you allow an extra 10 to 12 minutes into your morning routine and do them before jumping into the shower, and do them daily, over time you will get into better and better shape. These won't transform your body in a few weeks into Ms. Buffbody. However, done consistently over time will get and keep you in excellent physical condition.

Exercise is *incredibly* important in recovering from Fibromyalgia.

In fact, I would say that it is not possible to fully recover without some kind of regular, routine exercise.

The problem is that because we feel pain and/or fatigue, exercise is probably one of the last things we feel like doing.

But this really is where you will need to pull yourself up by the ole bootstraps and get yourself to do it. You will see that it does help.

Just remember, that no matter what form of exercise you do, start very light and build in intensity and duration very, very gradually.

Other forms of exercise that I would recommend are: swimming, light cardio workout on a good elliptical machine, yoga and pilates – but done very lightly and building up slowly.

Posture and Breathing

There are numerous factors regarding the ergonomics of how we sleep, work and carry our bodies that can have some very drastic effects on our bodies.

I really had no idea how much of an impact, but I consider this of great importance. Please bear with me while I expand on this and give some examples so I can convey to you how vital this is and how much of a connection this has to your pain levels.

I have had upper back and neck pain for years and I always assumed it was the top of my list of FM symptoms and that this was just the way it was.

Well, I have also had a bad habit of hunching over when I work at my computer.

I use a MacBook Air, which I love, but it does sit low on the table and you pretty much have to hunch over and bend your head downward to work on it. For the longest time I didn't realize how much pain this was causing in my neck and shoulders.

After reading something about this, I tried something that made a huge difference. My husband set me up with a large computer monitor on top of a stand and plugged my laptop into it. He then connected a keyboard and mouse and I started using a chair that had good ergonomics and great back support. Next thing I knew I was sitting up straight working away comfortably on my computer.

The result? After a few days my pain level drastically reduced and it made a huge difference.

When I was traveling I went back to using just my laptop and right away I notice the strain this puts on my neck and upper back within a few days, so this definitely is a factor.

Now I have a smaller, easily portable, wireless keyboard and mouse that I take with me when I travel so I can prop the laptop up on a box to put it at eye level and keep my back straight.

A mattress that doesn't offer good back support can be another big factor, as is your sleep position. For example, sleeping on your stomach and twisting your neck all night can also cause stiff and painful neck muscles.

High heel shoes or shoes that are too tight, uncomfortable or that have no arch support can also affect how you stand and not only cause foot and leg pain but can also cause back pain and problems.

Finally, I want to tell you one last story about posture and pain. All my life I never had any lower back problems or pain. I had a lot of neck and upper back pain, but not in my lower back. A couple of years ago I was working on learning some Pilates routines and the instructor talked about the position of your pelvis and the importance of tucking your pelvis in to strengthen your core. This was something that seemed to make sense to me, so I worked on it and over time changed my posture so that my pelvis was tucked in when I walked, stood and laid on my back.

Within several months of this I started to develop lower back problems. At the time, we were traveling and living in Baja Mexico and I attributed it to our mattress, which wasn't very good. However, getting a new mattress didn't change anything. I started trying various stretches and exercises and that didn't stop it either. One night I woke up in serious pain. I got up and tried to walk to the kitchen but only made it halfway before I was screaming in pain. My husband came rushing out to help me. The pain was so severe that it was too much for my body to handle. I was blacking out and vomiting.

My husband rushed me to the hospital.

They thought it was kidney stones, so I ended up going by ambulance up to a hospital in San Diego. It wasn't kidney stones after all but it was two herniated discs in my lower back. One disc had ruptured and leaked onto the nerves causing excruciating pain.

I ended up at a spine center in LA and was able to treat it without surgery to get it calmed down. Nevertheless, it continued to be painful and problematic for another year despite chiropractic treatments, physical therapy, massage, back exercises, traction and decompression treatments, ultrasound, laser, etc., etc., until I finally discovered the correct underlying cause – it was *my posture change!*

There is a woman named Esther Gokhale who experienced a similar lower back problem to the one I had. She also tried all kinds of remedies and finally ended up getting surgery.

When it flared up again, she decided to do some extensive research. I ran across an article about her and what she found. She has a website: **http://gokhalemethod.com/** and a book entitled *8 Steps to a Pain-free Back*. She also has a YouTube channel with a bunch of videos, but most of those videos are also on her website.

Needless to say, I think she hit the nail on the head and the simple posture changes that she recommends completely handled my lower back pain. It wasn't instant, but within a few weeks it really changed.

Realize that there are false ideas around that are pushed off as "good" or "correct posture" that just aren't. So, I would definitely recommend at least watching a couple of Gokhale's videos.

Correct posture can make a huge difference in your chronic pain levels.

So it's worth looking into and correcting. It could be the sofa you sit on to watch some TV in the evening sinks down and puts your back or neck in a bad position, or it could be a multitude of different things.

Now that you are aware of this, consider it throughout your day and make sure you have good posture and good ergonomics in chairs or other furniture that you use.

Diet and Nutrition, The Basics

Water:

First and foremost in this category is to drink a healthy amount of water each day.

Your body is more than 50% water, often between 60 and 70%. The percent of water depends on your hydration level. People feel thirsty when they have already lost around 2-3% of their body's water. Mental performance and physical coordination start to become impaired before thirst kicks in, typically around 1% dehydration. So, don't only drink water when you are thirsty, just drink and drink and drink water throughout the day thirsty or not.

It is very important to drink water that is not treated with fluoride or chlorine or other chemicals.

A reverse osmosis water purifier is a one-time

investment that you can install in your kitchen for drinking or cooking that is very well worth it.

If you don't like drinking plain water, then there are many things you can do to keep your body hydrated and keep mental and physical performance high. You can put lime or lemon juice in your water or sparkling water with the added benefits of helping to cleanse your liver, balancing pH levels and making it tastier.

You could make green tea with the added benefit of antioxidants. Sweeten it with Stevia and add lemon to improve the taste and not increase blood sugar. During warm weather, put it in the fridge and drink it iced.

For more information about Stevia, see http://www.healthkick.info/sugar-sweeteners/ . During warm weather, put it in the fridge and drink it iced.

Try drinking water first thing in the morning as

well as before each meal.

Keep water at your desk, in your car, in your purse, by your bed – make it easily accessible and sip on it throughout the day!

Vegetables: particularly green and leafy ones and colorful veggies are what you want to add into your diet as much as you can. Raw veggies are best and steamed is next best.

I also want to put a plug in here for organic. The amount of pesticides and dangerous chemicals that are used to grow a lot of our produce is astounding. Being ill to begin with, means that we certainly don't need to be shoveling more toxins into our body.

There is much more information on this and other important aspects of clean, healthy living in my book, *HealthKick, Easy Health Living Hacks.*

If you are not able to buy all organic produce

due to cost or availability, at least know that there are certain fruits and veggies that are more important to buy organic than others. There are certain ones that tend to absorb more of these pesticides than others. The "Dirty Dozen" are those vegetables and fruits that have been found to have the highest levels of pesticide contamination. Here's the list: **http://www.healthkick.info/clean-15-dirty-dozen/**

I used to work on dieting a lot. I have tried many, many diets. I lost weight with some but usually put it back on within weeks or months. With some, I found it very hard to lose anything. So I finally took a different approach. Instead of restricting myself, I decided to just work on eating more of the right things. One thing that stood out to me across all of the diets I have done was that veggies were almost always part of what was good to eat, especially green leafy veggies.

There wasn't one diet that said you couldn't eat veggies or that you had to restrict the amount of them that you could consume.

So I just started working more and more veggies into my life, mostly raw. I didn't restrict myself on what I could eat. I just focused on increasing my intake of veggies. The reverse psychology worked really well. I started eating less and less carbs and sugars. It calmed my appetite down, and my overall portions of food were smaller. I had more energy and was more able to get in some exercise.

I did the same with my husband. He's not a big dieter. He's one of those guys that was blessed for most of his life – able to eat anything he wanted and never gained weight. However, once he hit middle age the party was over. Over time he put on 40 pounds.

Now we are both gradually coming down on

our weight and exercising more – just by simply following the fundamentals covered here in this chapter.

Here are some ways I have worked more veggies into my daily routine that made it easy to eat them more often:

- Veggie smoothies – I make these in my blender to still get all of the fiber (as opposed to juicing). I use spinach, kale, avocado and 4-5 cups of water as a base. I then add different fruit combinations such as strawberries or a berry medley, mango, pineapple/coconut, kiwi fruit and green apples, etc. I add some Stevia and blend really well. They taste great and I love them. My husband slurps them down too and that's saying a lot. The fruit and Stevia sweeten the drink up and you would be surprised by how good it tastes. There are literally tons of recipes for these if you do a Google search, not to mention books on Amazon.

- Veggie snack plates – There are easy. Just get a bag of those baby carrots, some celery, cucumbers and some broccoli. Chop up the celery, cucumbers and broccoli. Arrange them on a plate and put some reduced fat cream cheese in the center. Have them in the fridge or put them out on the counter at snack time. Chomp on these when you get those afternoon and evening hunger pangs.
- Salads – If you make a great tasting salad (that is creative and tasty), then make enough to last you (and anyone else that you are feeding) for two days of lunch and dinner. Then you can eat salad as part of lunch and dinner as the first course. You get your raw veggies in and you help curb your appetite to be able to eat smaller portions of the rest of the meal.

- Snack packs to take to work or on the go – baby carrots and other chopped veggies (celery, cucumber, etc.) and fruits – make a bunch of packs at once in Ziploc bags so that they are easy to grab and take with you when you are rushing to get to work or wherever.
- Juicing – Once a week I will usually do a big batch of juice. It is so rich in nutrients and very alkalizing for the body. The mean green juice recipe is what I use.

Low sugar fruits: These make great snacks and after dinner desserts. I particularly like all berries, cantaloupe, watermelon, nectarines, papaya, apples and peaches.

Nuts, seeds and beans: Nuts and seeds that are raw are also a great snack or are good to use in salads. Beans and lentils are high in protein and fiber and slow burning carbs.

Some whole grains: Whole sprouted grains

being the best and most nutritious. Avoid or cut back on wheat flour and gluten as much as possible.

Fats: It is very important to stay clear of trans fats as they can be very damaging. The oils I recommend you use are virgin coconut oil for baking, frying or whatever, organic butter, extra virgin olive oil or avocado oil (these last two should not be used at very high temperatures). You need to watch for trans fats that are added into other foods, such as crackers, chips and tons of other things. Anything that says "shortening", "partially hydrogenated vegetable oil" or "hydrogenated vegetable oil" contains trans fat. Most margarine contains trans fats.

Stay away from fast food or processed foods.

As you eat more and more of the nutritious foods I have listed above, it should be easier and come somewhat naturally to eat less sugar and simple carbohydrates. This is important because if consumed in excess as sugar and carbs will rob you of already lacking and badly needed energy in your cells. They appear to give you energy at first by shooting your blood sugar up, but then here comes the heavy load of insulin that bombs your blood sugar into a low-energy ditch.

You will likely crave sugars and/or simple carbs when you are tired or in pain and you can get a very short-lived pleasure from consuming them. However, matters just get worse after that and you can end up feeling even more tired or experience more pain. If you can break away from them and stay away from them, then your energy levels will build back up.

Protein: Low mercury fish and shellfish that are not farm raised, as well as chicken and turkey breast meat that are free of hormones and antibiotics, are great sources of protein. Eggs are as well. I also often make a protein shake each day using all natural plant based protein powder that has no added sweeteners in it. I add some berries and some liquid minerals.

Meats and Dairy: If you can buy organic meats and fowl, this is definitely best. You can often get some decent deals at Costco. However, if you cannot buy organic, at least avoid meats, pork, chicken and turkey, as well as eggs and milk products that have been raised with the use of antibiotics and hormones.

There is not that much price difference for this. Chicken and turkey meats and eggs in particular are much more readily available to buy in most supermarkets without antibiotics or hormones.

Many dishes that are routinely made with ground beef can be made with ground turkey meat instead. Spaghetti, meatloaf, lasagna, chili and even tacos can be made with ground turkey and you can hardly taste the difference.

As for meats, organic beef is becoming more and more available and really is recommended. If you are going to buy regular beef (not hormone and antibiotic free), at least try to avoid beef that is higher in fat content, such as ribeye steak, ground chuck or pork.

Regular bacon, because it is so high in fat, is one of the worst. Most of the bad stuff is stored in the fat, so go for lean meats.

Canadian bacon or turkey bacon can replace regular bacon as trying to get hormone and anti-biotic free bacon is usually obscenely expensive. I've tried numerous brands of turkey bacon. From my point of view some are pretty icky and some can be quite nice. If you try it and don't like it, then try another brand before you give up on it.

I have generally tried to only eat red meat once per week and when I do it is only grass fed, without hormones or antibiotics.

As such meats tend to be more expensive, I have opted for chicken and turkey much more often.

Avoid pre-packaged deli meats or processed meats (hot dogs, sausage, lunch meats). Unless you buy organic, these are heavily processed using preservatives and colorants and will use meats or fowl that have been raised using hormones and antibiotics. The best is to buy enough of your meats to be able to slice some off or use leftovers for sandwiches or to use with salads for lunches.

Good alternatives to milk are coconut milk and almond milk. Make sure you get the unsweetened kind and preferably organic.

Canned Foods and Plastic Bottles: Nearly all canned foods of any kind have a lining inside the can that contains BPA-containing resin (BPA stands for Bisphenol A, a carbon-based synthetic compound).

Plastic water bottles should also be checked to make sure they do not contain BPA. Once you check your brand, you can usually just stick to that brand.

BPA has been linked to various health issues, including thyroid malfunctions, obesity, cancer and reproductive problems. There is a lot of controversy on the subject and various investigations underway.

So, I recommend avoiding as much BPA as possible. This is particularly important for infants or young children as well as pregnant women. In short, avoid use of canned foods where possible. Sauces are often available in glass containers. Never cook or microwave in plastic or Styrofoam containers.

Sugars and Sweeteners: Cutting out sugar was tough but very rewarding because I was addicted. Sugar would steal my energy. I might feel good for a bit right after eating it, but soon afterward I would slump. If I did a major sugar binge, then I would often feel really bad that night and/or the next day. Sometimes it would even cause a full flare that lasted a couple of days. It was hard to get off of sugar and took weeks before I was use to it, but life is so much better without it. I have much more energy.

For more information on nutrition and easy ways to live healthier, I have written another book entitled *HealthKick: Easy Life Hacks for Healthier Living*. It has a lot more great tips and easy ways to work in healthy habits and routines. I really highly recommend it. It is packed with great and usable information that is particularly needed if you are suffering from chronic illness.

It will be available on Amazon. And you can visit www.HealthKick.info and sign up for the blog posts to stay up-to-date on great healthy living tips.

Supplements – What Can Be Beneficial

I have shelves and shelves of different vitamins, minerals, herbs, amino acids and other supplements that I have tried over the years. I must admit, most of them didn't seem to make a damn bit of difference.

Here is what I finally concluded and the supplements that I now take regularly.

Minimally, I always recommend that you take basic vitamins – A to E, including higher dosages of B vitamins (like a couple B 100s per day), C (at least 1,000 mg per day), D3 5000 to 10,000 IU per day and E. Vitamin D deficiencies have been linked to FMS and other auto-immune diseases.

B and D vitamins particularly have been found to be deficient in those who suffer from Fibromyalgia.

I found that B vitamins helped ease depression. Also, low D3 has been linked to Fibromyalgia.

Several months ago I switched to a liquid vitamin and mineral supplement that is so much easier to take and I think it works better. This is likely because of the fact that these come from natural sources as opposed to being synthetic, resulting in better absorption. One capful daily is super easy to take. I recommend one that is made from natural organic sources – mainly fruits and vegetables. You can still take a couple extra supplements that you want to boost in addition to the liquid. For years I took a lot of vitamins and minerals in pill form daily – this is so much easier and it seems to work so much better!

Get one that you like the taste of. I have tried several and I noticed that the ones that taste bad get harder and harder to get down your throat.

This one is what I use and it is the best I have found. The link below gives info on it. You can buy it on Amazon. It tastes pretty good: **http://naturalvitality.com/organic-life-vitamins/**

You may find other better options than this. I have not done enough research to be able to tell you what is best but I do know vitamins help a lot so take the time to find what works for you.

Probiotics are also really important. I have covered more information on probiotics later in this book in the chapter on the immune system.

Minerals and trace minerals that include selenium, molybdenum, potassium and manganese.

Additional calcium to help prevent osteoarthritis and magnesium can often help with the achy muscles.

I use liquid minerals that include trace minerals and I just put a capful in a protein drink each day.

I usually supplement my diet with a daily protein drink. I use an organic plant based protein powder that has no added sugar or sweeteners except for stevia. I usually make a drink with some organic fruit, water, liquid minerals and a scoop or two of protein powder. It tastes like a yummy milkshake, is filling and is a way to increase my protein without a lot of carbs.

Hydrolyzed Collagen, Glucosamine, Chondroitin, MSM and hyaluronic acid all can help joint pain. There are some powdered forms you can get that have all of this. I just throw a scoop of this in my daily protein drink and I can't even taste the difference.

Melatonin – as needed to help with sleep as covered in the chapter on sleep.

Omega 3 oils are also extremely important.

Turmeric, a spice you can use in cooking (it is the key spice in curry) and you can get in capsule form, can be very helpful for relieving inflammation.

Viruses and Infectious Diseases Can Be Causing Many of Your Symptoms

This is the section that I consider one of the most VITAL to recovery.

Addressing viruses and infectious diseases made a HUGE difference for me, many times over.

When I refer to infectious diseases, this includes bacterial, viral and fungal/yeast infections.

Because most of the features of Chronic Fatigue Syndrome, Fibromyalgia and Lupus resemble those of a lingering viral illness, a number of researchers, doctors and treatment centers have gone in the direction that a virus or some other infectious agent plays a major role in the cause of these syndromes.

There are several books and research studies on the connection between viral, bacterial and fungal infections and FMS/CFS as well as Lyme and Lupus, some of which I will list with links and quotes throughout this chapter. For additional references to sources of information, you can go to the books that I recommend in this chapter and you can do your own further research as you wish.

It is already well known that Lyme disease comes from a bacterial infection as a result of being bitten by a tick carrying one of several strains. There are other studies that show that Chlamydia Pneumoniae, an infectious bacterium, has been implicated in a number of these illnesses.

Chronic Fatigue Syndrome, Fibromyalgia and other autoimmune disease patients are often found with elevated levels of antibodies, meaning their body's immune system is fighting some form of infection.

When diagnosed, such infections can end up including those that cause Lyme disease, Candida (yeast infection), herpes virus type 6 (HHV-6), human T cell lymph tropic virus (HTLV), Epstein-Barr, measles, coxsackie B, cytomegalovirus, or parvovirus.

You can read more about this on the Envita Clinic's website here: **http://goo.gl/L5Y9m**

In other words, these major syndromes and diseases can have a host of co-infections that have brought about immunological, hormonal, and neuroendocrine changes.

There are a number of studies that have found that these kinds of viral and bacterial infections can cause actual alterations in genes and these genetic alterations often impact the immune function, intracellular communication and energy transfer.

I recommend the Envita because it is a clinic in Scottsdale Arizona that specializes in advanced integrative medicine treating a broad range of conditions using the latest scientific technologies and approaches. Their focus is on cancer, Lyme disease, FMS, CFS and other autoimmune diseases.

They address underlying viruses and infectious diseases as part of their protocol. They say that CFS is sometimes even referred to as "Chronic Fatigue Immune Dysfunction Syndrome" because many cases studies of CFS patients have detected immune system irregularities.

Envita states that almost 100% of the time they find decreased key immune function in CFS patients by running the correct diagnostics. For more information and other interesting articles on the subject, you can go to: **http://www.envita.com**

Another study regarding the use of an antiviral protocol was presented at a recent American College of Rheumatology annual meeting.

The results were very promising. A study of 143 Fibromyalgia patients that followed a specific antiviral regimen concluded the following:

"A proprietary combination of famciclovir, which we postulate is inhibiting herpesvirus replication, and celecoxib, known to inhibit both herpesvirus replication and reactivation, was efficacious in treating multiple symptoms of FM. Given the simultaneous improvement in many domains and the surprising tolerability of this combination of drugs, we believe this combination warrants further study as a potential new therapy for fibromyalgia patients."

You can read more about it here.
http://www.healthcentral.com/chronic-pain/c/5949/173154/fibromyalgia-promising/

A further good source of information on this topic is a book entitled *The New Fibromyalgia Remedy, Stop your pain now with a new antiviral regimen,* by Daniel C. Dantini MD. Here he suggests that antiviral medicine and food allergy treatment can be very effective in treating FMS. Dr. Dantini documents links between Fibromyalgia and several viruses, particularly the Epstein-Barr virus, cytomegalovirus, herpes virus 6 and/or parvovirus. He says antiviral medications work in 70 to 75 % of his patients, along with allergy and sensitivities treatments, massage and other therapies.

Using Dantini's treatment method, most patients see their symptoms improve by "about 20 to 50 percent during the first four weeks," the book says.

Most people take the antiviral medications for 10 to 14 weeks, while others need the drugs for up to six months.

Throughout the book, there are patient success stories as well as data samples, references, and appendices that provide clinical details.

It would seem that these very common viral infections have the ability to stay within the human body unnoticed for years. In fact, the majority of the population probably has a number of like entities in their system. However, for those of us that suffer with Fibromyalgia, CFS and other similar conditions, these infections get triggered and attack the system again and again with each new flare up.

With a compromised or overworked immune system, other bacterial or fungal infections can develop more easily as the body's defenses are in a weakened state, making things even worse.

Further, although I have largely talked about viruses, however bacterial infections, such as Chlamydia Pneumoniae, and yeast infections such as Candida, can also be major or at least partial culprits.

Candida, short for Candidiasis, an overgrowth of a type of yeast in the digestive tract, can also cause many similar symptoms, including fatigue, IBS, compromised immune system, cognitive problems, genito-urinary infections, arthritis-like symptoms, food and chemical allergies, MS-like symptoms and more.

It is not uncommon for Candida to flare-up after a round of antibiotics, as while the antibiotics kill the bad bacteria causing infection, it also kills the good bacteria in your body that is a vital part of your immune system, allowing yeast/fungal infection overgrowth throughout the digestive tract.

In summary, based on the extensive amount of materials on the subject that I have studied and on my own experience, there is no doubt in my mind that Fibromyalgia and Chronic Fatigue as well as Lupus and Lyme disease are related diseases that involve viral/bacterial/yeast infection or multiple infections, followed by an exaggerated defense reaction by the body.

I sincerely believe that it is a matter of finding a doctor who is competent and a bit more cutting edge in the fields of virology and infectious diseases. Dr. Dantini's book lists a number of such doctors. If you find one who will do the appropriate testing to discover these and then follow a real treatment protocol, then you too may have a miraculous recovery.

I saw many doctors and tried many treatments, none of which gave any lasting resolution to my symptoms. It was very disheartening. As time went on, the pain and fatigue took its toll, combined with the despair that I may never be well again. This all changed when I went to a doctor who was a specialist is virology and infectious diseases.

My tests showed that I had a type of walking pneumonia (Chlamydia Pneumoniae), Epstein-Barr Virus, HHV6 and Candida.

It is also likely I had contracted Lyme disease from a tick bite that caused a serious rash when I was younger.

Wow! First of all, the fact that someone found <u>something</u> that actually made sense was a ray of hope that there may be a resolution.

I started on a program of standard treatments and started to feel <u>dramatically</u> better within a couple of months, which was nothing short of a miracle to me!

I took a longer round of antibiotics to address the pneumonia, along with eating a lot of yogurt and taking high quality probiotics throughout and afterwards (particularly as I already had a yeast overgrowth in my gut and antibiotics would make matters worse).

I then followed an antiviral regimen using Valacyclovir, which I took for a couple of months. Lastly, I followed a protocol to handle the yeast overgrowth with a specific diet, an anti-fungal regimen and replacing the good bacteria in my gut with probiotics.

I GOT BETTER! I FELT GOOD! I was able to go back to work full-time.

My husband and I started our own small marketing firm and grew it into a steady, thriving company. I got my life back! So, I am convinced that you can too!

You should work with a doctor knowledgeable in viral and infectious diseases and get properly tested – a complete viral panel as well as other more common infectious diseases including common bacterial and fungal infections found to be connected with these syndromes.

The appropriate antiviral and/or antibiotic or

antifungal medications will likely be administered to treat what is found, all under that doctor's care and supervision.

My main doctor, Marcus Spurlock MD of Dallas Texas, was fantastic.

He is very experienced in the field of viral disease and is a specialist in treating Fibromyalgia and CFS.

His practice is Renewed Vitality, located in Dallas, TX, **www.renewedvitalitymd.com**.

Once you have done an initial visit and exam with Dr. Spurlock, he will also perform additional appointments by phone if you do not live nearby. You can get any lab-work that he orders done at a lab in your own local area.

Dr. Teitelbaum's book, *From Fatigued to Fantastic*, is excellent and I highly recommend it. Jacob Teitelbaum, M.D. is the director of The Annapolis Center for Effective

CFS/Fibromyalgia Therapies and his website is **http://www.endfatigue.com/**. He also does consultations by phone.

Dr. Rodger Murphee is another excellent resource, along with his book *Treating and Beating Fibromyalgia and Chronic Fatigue Syndrome*. Much more information is available on his website and blog: **http://drrodgermurphree.com/**

There is also Envita, a highly recommended clinic located in Scottsdale, Arizona.

Dr. Dantini practices on the east coast of Florida.

If you are near any of these clinics or are willing to make a trip, then I would recommend them. If not, then you will need to do some research and talk to your PCP about options of specialists that you could see that are near you.

Stabilizing Your Improvements

Once I had been under treatment long enough to get back on my feet, I was able to start working again and taking care of things around the house. When I completed my treatment, I had my life pretty much back to normal. I was exercising daily, working, cooking, doing housework, etc. Life was good again and stayed good for a couple of years.

Then I went through a period of very serious stress. A situation blew up and both my husband and I were engaged in handling something that was very, very stressful, and which went on for several months. I was still physically okay through much of it, but then finally it happened – I had a huge relapse. Heavy pain, horrible fatigue and a lot of despair once again swept into my life.

I knew I had to bring the stress to an end and we did.

After resolving that situation, I went back to my doctor. He explained to me some very important points:

a. Heavy stress is a huge load on one's body and stress alone can trigger Fibromyalgia.

b. The type of pneumonia that I had had was a kind of nanobacteria that can be quite hard to kill. Sometimes if you don't thoroughly nuke it out, you can relapse.

c. These types of viral infections that I had actually stay in your body, just like chicken pox or other known viruses, but the body usually develops defenses to them and can hold them at bay and keep them dormant. However, if for some reason your defenses are down (such as a period of heavy stress, an accident, etc.) and your immune system is somehow compromised, then these viruses can reactivate, just like shingles can suddenly hit with someone who contracted chickenpox when they were young – it's the same virus reactivating.

d. My immune system was and had been in a weakened state and I would need to work to build it back up and strengthen it if I ever wanted to stably keep these viruses and infectious diseases in a dormant state.

So, once again I followed the same protocol that I had the first time. And once again it worked, just like it had the first time. Over the next couple of years I had to do a fair amount of traveling. We rented our house out and lived for short periods in several different countries where my husband was doing work-related projects. The first time it worked out okay, but each subsequent trip resulted in another relapse of my symptoms.

In addition to the travel itself, there were other factors – diet changes, quality of mattresses, quality of water and even air and other factors – that ended up being triggers for flares or partial relapses.

Finally, my doctor suggested that I go onto a lower dose of the antiviral and just take it everyday while I was traveling and possibly even for the rest of my life. I did that for quite some time and it seemed to help, although after a long travel I often had to go back onto a full dose for a short while. Even though there were some advantages to being on antivirals, like almost never getting the flu, I knew there were some long-term use side effects that could hurt my kidneys, liver, digestive tract and my immune system. So I started researching alternatives.

A recent study done on FMS and CFS uncovered some important information regarding our immune system.

The results from this study are summarized in an article by Dr. Teitelbaum. In short, this article states that a recent study of those with FMS and CFS showed widespread changes and deficiencies in the immune system.

Work by Dr. Mark Sivieri in Maryland also found that there are deficiencies in critical antibodies that may be contributing to immune dysfunction in FMS and CFS patients.

One very expensive treatment that is getting some very good results is intravenous gamma globulin, mostly used with patients who are so sick that they are bedridden and do not respond to other treatments. Gamma globulin can cost as much as $50,000 per year and is very difficult to get covered by insurance.

Because most of us don't have an extra 50K to spend on this treatment, I dug deeper to find more treatments that could be followed and afforded.

Low and behold, I found a whole new world of natural solutions to the problem. It was like the last part of the puzzle finally falling into place!

A Drug-free, Natural Approach to Treatment

Once you isolate and treat any infectious diseases with appropriate medications under a doctor's care, there are then VITAL steps you will need to take to stabilize and better your improvement. Or maybe you want to forego the drug regimens completely and go the naturopathic route solely. This is something that you and your doctor can decide.

I've known that there were supplements and even some foods that were helpful for the immune system, such as garlic, certain mushrooms, zinc, etc., but I wasn't so sure about natural treatments that could actually kill viruses and shorten the duration of the illnesses caused by viruses. Well, after some digging, I found quite a few resources available that have antiviral, antibacterial and antifungal properties – some of them are herbs, but not all.

I'll give a brief summary of what I have found and in some cases will include some links to further research and information.

The natural supplements described here could be a way to keep viruses dormant and deal with infections. Some of these are promising but really have not been subject to thorough clinical trials. Therefore, don't get stuck on using just one of these. Correct use of several antiviral products together with immune-boosting nutrients and vitamins and a healthy diet as covered in other chapters of this book is really the recommended route to take.

Once again, I want to stress the following: None of the health topics presented in this book or at **www.FibromyalgiaFree.org** have been evaluated or approved by the FDA. They should not replace personal judgment or medical treatment when indicated, nor are they intended to diagnose, treat, cure, or prevent any disease.

Always talk to your doctor or naturopathic physician about the use of any of the recommendations for diet, supplements, drugs, exercise or any other complimentary modalities. Here is a list, along with a bit of info on each, of what I have gotten the best results from:

Fulvic Acid:

Fulvic acid is a humic extract (humic is the major organic constituents of soil [humus] which is produced by biodegradation of dead organic matter). Fulvic acid is mineral complex found in rich organic humus soil and also certain ancient plant deposits. Many medical studies show that humic substances, especially fulvic acid, have the power to protect against cancer AND other viruses.

Some studies have even shown reversal of cancers, tumors and viruses using special humic substance therapies.

Many studies and extensive references exist, a few of which are referenced on my website here: **fibromyalgiafree.org/fulvic-acid-antiviral-and-fibromyalgia/**

I take 1 ounce of fulvic acid daily. It is easy to take in liquid form with a very mild taste. I pour 1 ounce into a small glass each day and take a sip or two three times a day.

Zinc:

Zinc has been tested in trials and proven to reduce the duration and severity of cold symptoms.

Topical application of zinc has also been used to treat cold sores, which are caused by the herpes simplex virus. One study found that using zinc monoglycerolate resulted in complete healing of cold sore lesions in 70% of subjects, whereas zinc oxide only healed 9%. So the form of zinc used is also important.

Olive Leaf:

The olive leaves contain elenoic acid, which has been identified as a potent inhibitor of a wide range of viruses in laboratory tests. The calcium salt of elenoic acid destroyed all of the viruses it was tested against, including influenza, herpes, polio and coxsackie viruses.

A clinical trial in Budapest involving over 500 patients concluded that olive leaf extract was extremely effective in treating a wide range of viruses and infections. Fast recovery as a result of taking the extract was noted in 115 out of 119 patients with respiratory tract infections and 120 out of 172 patients with viral infections.

Lomatium:

The antiviral and antibacterial properties of Lomatium dissectum are utilized in the treatment of some of the most difficult viral diseases and may be part of a protocol in the treatment of Hepatitis-C, Influenza, HIV, AIDS, Chronic-Fatigue, pneumonia, bronchitis, herpes simplex, sinusitis, and common colds.

When used on a group of patients with Hepatitis C, it resulted in dramatic reductions in viral counts. It has been used for other viral syndromes, flu, upper respiratory illness and sinusitis with good results.

Garlic:

Garlic has been used for more than 5000 years and hailed for its medicinal properties dating back to the days of the pharaohs. In laboratory studies, garlic was found to possess antiviral, antibacterial and antifungal properties.

One of its most important compounds is allicin, which produces garlic's pungent odor. Aged garlic contains very little allicin, so it is important to use fresh garlic.

Allicin and various other sulfur compounds in fresh garlic can be used successfully to treat the common cold virus, various strains of influenza viruses and herpes simplex virus types I and II.

So eat as much garlic as you can and you can take high quality garlic capsules.

Goldenseal:

Goldenseal is a fantastic antiviral. It contains berberine, which can kill off too much of your natural intestinal flora, so it is recommended to take this for one week and then take a week off while you take more probiotics before resuming. You can also often get Goldenseal and Echinacea together in capsules or tinctures.

Echinacea:

The herb echinacea (Echinacea Purpurea) is one of the better-known herbs for supporting the immune system.

Roots and flowering portions of the plant have been found to help reduce the duration and severity of colds, bronchial and upper respiratory infections in clinical trials and may have direct antiviral properties.

Elderberry:

Black elderberry has antiviral properties. One clinical trial showed improvement in 90% of patients of influenza symptoms and higher levels of influenza antibodies.

An independent study performed in Norway found elderberry helped to reduce the duration of influenza symptoms by about four days.

The activity of elderberry against other viral infections, including HIV and herpes, has also been found to completely inhibit the replication of four strains of herpes simplex virus, including two strains resistant to the drug acyclovir (Zovirax).

Liquorice:

The SARS (Severe Acute Respiratory Syndrome) epidemic many years ago spurred the search for active antiviral compounds to treat the disease. Researchers at the Institute of Medical Virology at Frankfurt tested four pharmaceutical drugs (including ribavirin, the recommended treatment) and glycyrrhizin, a compound found in the root of the liquorice plant on SARS patients. The published results found that glycyrrhizin out-performed all four drugs in inhibiting the virus. It was also non-toxic to virus-infected cells. Liquorice has also shown qualities of inhibiting the reproduction of HIV in lab studies.

Clinical trials have shown that injections of glycyrrhizin may have a beneficial effect on AIDS with some evidence that orally administered liquorice also may be safe and effective for long-term treatment of HIV infection.

A preliminary trial involving people with acute and chronic viral hepatitis found that taking 2 ½ grams of liquorice three times a day (containing 750 mg glycyrrhizin) was superior to the antiviral drug inosine poly-IC. Entire liquorice extract (not de-glycyrrhizinated liquorice or DGL) may be a very effective treatment for other viral illnesses.

Monolaurin:

Monolaurin is a chemical made from lauric acid, which is found in coconut milk and breast milk. Monolaurin is often used by Naturopaths for preventing and treating colds (the common cold), flu (influenza), swine flu, herpes, shingles, and other infections.

It is also used to treat chronic fatigue syndrome (CFS) and to boost the immune system. Monolaurin has antibacterial, antiviral, and other antimicrobial effects *in vitro*. It has not really been tested or proven on humans.

Mushrooms:

There are a number of mushrooms that are renown for their antiviral and antimicrobial attributes. Maitake, Shiitake and Reishi are some of the most well known ones, but there are others.

You can get mushroom capsules that have combinations of these immune system boosting mushrooms, and you can add these mushrooms into foods you prepare as much as possible.

Pau D'Arco:

Comes from the inner bark of the tree which contains a high proportion of chemicals called quinoids, including the compound lapachol, which has been found in laboratory tests to be active against various viruses, including herpes simplex types I and II, influenza, polio virus and others.

St John's Wort:

In addition to being a well-known remedy for depression and easing pain, some lab studies have found that St. John's Wort also has antiviral properties against influenza, herpes simplex and HIV.

Colloidal Silver:

A colloid is a suspension of ultra-fine particles that neither dissolve nor settle out, even with changes in concentration. It is thought to work by interfering with the enzymes that enable viruses, bacteria and fungi to utilize oxygen so it basically suffocates them. Many case studies have indicated that the use of various forms of colloidal silver dramatically reduced the activity of the viruses and cleared up bacterial infections in patients.

There are reports of the successful use of colloidal silver to fight the hepatitis C virus.

There is also a fair amount of controversy about colloidal silver with some reports saying it has no effect. It did seem to help on bacterial infections including topically.

Lemon, Lime, Lemon Balm, Cinnamon, Peppermint And Basil Essential Oils:

These all have some antiviral attributes. There is more info in an excellent article here: **http://www.sustainablebabysteps.com/antiviral-essential-oils.html**

If you don't like taking a bunch of different things, then here is a supplement called Ultimate Immunity, made by Nature's Way, that has a nice combination of supplements in it that are great for strengthening your immune system.

You can get it on Amazon.

The following ones listed here I have not tried, but are reported to have anti-viral properties:

Oil Of Oregano:

Another serious antiviral and antioxidant, you can take oil oregano internally (1-4 drops in water twice a day) when indicated on the bottle, or externally on affected skin.

Apparently, you can also cook with it, although I have never tried this.

Clove Essential Oil:

One of the most potent of antiviral essential oils. It's a strong antiseptic as well as antifungal oil. It's great for cleaning with its antibacterial/disinfectant attributes. To use topically, dilute with two parts carrier oil. Some say it can be taken internally with the right precautions.

Helichrysum Essential Oil:

This oil is powerfully antiviral, as well as antibacterial, and it can be used to treat muscle spasms.

Most people can take it undiluted and it is generally recognized as safe to consume when indicated.

Melaleuca Essential Oil:

Also an excellent antiviral essential oil, in addition to being antifungal, antibacterial and can be used to treat parasites. Some of these will work better than others for each individual, so I really recommend your own trial and error until you find what produces the most improvement.

Again, I must stress that I am not prescribing or telling you to take any of these supplements, herbs or oils. I strongly recommend that you find a good naturopath or holistic doctor to advise you on what to take, how to take it, dosages, etc. I am not a doctor. I am not a certified nutritionist. I am only telling you what I have found in my research and what I have tried myself that helped me.

I do not recommend any long-term use of internally taken essential oils as there is some evidence that it can overtax your liver.

Please use every caution. I could not bear the thought of any harmful effects caused to anyone as a result of incorrect use of these supplements. Consult a professional. If you experience any bad side effects from taking a supplement, immediately stop and consult a professional.

Additional Steps to Build a Strong Immune System

Along with any drug or supplement regimens you may choose, it is very important to follow a program to strengthen your immune system as much as possible.

Many of the natural supplements, herbs and oils listed in the previous chapter will also help to strengthen your immune system.

In addition to these, and from all of the research I have done, here is a summary of what I have gleaned as some of the most important steps to take in building a strong and robust immune system.

1. Probiotics are _vital_. I have found that raw probiotics are far more effective than the kind you buy off the shelf that is not live. In most health food stores you can find a refrigerated section of probiotics.

You want one that has many strains and are in the billions. I like Garden of Life.

If you just completed a round of antibiotics or you have been a frequent user of antibiotics, I would recommend that you do something intense for a short period to repopulate your gut with good bacteria as fast as possible to avoid an overgrowth of bad bacteria - something like Garden of Life Raw Probiotics 5-Day Max Care.

After that, you should go onto a regular daily dose that you always take just like daily vitamins. I also recommend taking them between meals or on an empty stomach.

2. Decrease toxic load into your body. That means no smoking, no pollution, no toxic chemicals ingested, inhaled or absorbed through your skin (cleaning agents, hair dye, etc.) See the chapter below on this subject to understand more about this.

3. Cut out all junk food, sugar, artificial sweeteners and processed foods. Make healthy choices and eat organic produce and meats as often as you can. Minimally follow the points laid out in my other book entitled *HealthKick, Easy Healthy Living Hacks*.

4. Drink a lot of water daily as well as green tea. Green tea has been considered a medicinal remedy in Chinese tradition for over 4000 years and its many health benefits have recently been validated by scientific methods. Green tea contains a group of flavonoids that appear to inhibit viral infections. Drink water that is free of fluoride, chlorine and other chemicals.

5. Get good sleep.

6. Testing for environmental and food allergies and sensitivities can also help. Allergies and sensitivities can overwork the immune system and weaken it.

The Important Role that Hormones Play

The body produces a number of hormones that, when produced in the correct balance, keep the body functioning normally. However, if the body produces too much or too little of even just one hormone, then this can affect the way the body functions and the way you feel.

Your endocrine system works sort of like an orchestra. Even one overactive or underactive hormone gland can have a cascade of effects.

Hormones are incredible chemical messengers in our body that affect our brain, heart, bones, muscles, and reproductive organs and are an essential part of the workings of every cell in the human body. Hormones work best when balanced, but they can become imbalanced.

Here's one little example – it's a story that makes a point about hormones.

Recently my shoulder started to get stiff and painful. Over a period of a few days it worsened so much so that I could hardly use my arm at all. I had a hard time getting to sleep, as it was so painful that I couldn't get comfortable enough and it would often wake me up once I did finally doze off.

I started researching to figure out what this was and concluded it was a condition called "frozen shoulder". This condition most often affects menopausal women. As I read up more and more about this condition, I got more and more freaked out. It can last a year. Painful physical therapy is most recommended. Most pain meds don't help it. I studied all of the top medical sites – Mayo Clinic, WebMD and others. It all just sounded absolutely horrible.

The thought of losing the use of my arm for a year and enduring this pain was more than depressing. Overall, it was looking pretty bleak.

So, I starting digging a lot deeper to find alternative treatments and stumbled upon a few obscure articles and some forums that talked about the relation of "frozen shoulder" to hormones. It made sense because this most often affects women in menopause. After reading everything I could find about it, I ended up slathered on some of my bio-identical hormone creams (both estrogen and progesterone).

By the time I woke up the next morning it was greatly improved, and I mean a LOT. By the following day it was completely back to normal.

Can you imagine going through a year of agony by not knowing that some hormones could handle the whole situation within a day or two? WOW!

That blew me away.

Not to mention the fact that I had also been experiencing more joint pain, and what do you know, it had everything to do with my estrogen levels dropping when I went into menopause.

Here is one article about it: **http://www.34-menopause-symptoms.com/joint-pain.htm** – see under "Causes of Joint Pain" section.

There is a somewhat common condition called estrogen dominance that can affect women. Even if your estrogen levels aren't that high, if your progesterone levels are very low (too low for the proper balance between the two), then you can still have estrogen dominance. I think some doctors are maybe a bit too fast to say estrogen dominance, but there are certainly women who have benefited greatly by an increase in progesterone that balanced out those hormones.

There is an excellent article on this that I recommend reading:

https://www.womentowomen.com/hormonal-health/estrogen-dominance/ - not only does it explain this is much more detail, along with symptoms, but it also explains several options of how to treat it.

Another example of hormone issues is that a number of studies on Chronic Fatigue Syndrome have shown that patients have lower cortisol levels, a stress hormone produced by the adrenal glands. It has been suggested that such cortisol deficiencies could be largely responsible for Chronic Fatigue Syndrome patients having impaired or weakened responses to psychological or physical stresses such as worry, infection, or exercise.

It is also quite common for those suffering from Fibromyalgia, CFS and other chronic illnesses to have low thyroid (hypothyroidism), low adrenal hormones – cortisol and DHEA – as well as low pregnenolone.

Rather than trying to explain each hormone and the varying issues that can occur with each, the best thing to do is to get complete hormone testing done.

Get proper hormone testing done through a qualified doctor and work to correct deficiencies or imbalances either through diet and lifestyle changes, natural supplements or prescribed bio-identical hormone replacement therapy.

It is recommended that any infections, viruses or yeast overgrowths be cleared up first before hormone replacement is begun. It is more effective and easier to monitor and gets everything properly balanced.

Using the Guaifenesin Protocol

R. Paul St. Amand, M.D. and Claudia Craig Marek run the Fibromyalgia Treatment Center in Los Angeles California. They co-authored a book entitled *What Your Doctor May Not Tell You About Fibromyalgia*. His goal was that someone could read the book and follow the protocol it laid out and get well.

I was one such patient who did come to see him after following the guidelines laid out in the book. After a couple of years of following these fairly simple procedures, I got so well that I decided that I no longer had Fibromyalgia – I was at that moment cured.

I won't tell you about the completely crazy and stupid things I did to my body after that (diving right back into a very high stress life because "I was all better now"), which caused a complete relapse of the condition.

However I will tell you that this is a treatment that seems to get a result, but it is something you need to continue to follow.

The theory it is based on is that FMS is caused by a metabolic defect resulting in retention of a biochemical substance within the cells themselves – a metabolic malfunction that results in an inability to produce energy.

These build up over years. The treatment involves taking an expectorant called Guaifenesin twice per day to purge this build up in the cells and reverse their effects.

There is a fair amount to the protocol, including eliminating all salicylates (plant products) from use on skin, including toothpaste, shampoo, soap, cosmetics, etc. This is not that hard as there are plenty of these types of products on the market without salicylates. However it does take a conscious effort to keep this point in.

It also requires that if one is hypoglycemic, that this be addressed with the appropriate diet.

There are also numerous articles that say the theory behind this protocol is unfounded. If you simply do a Google search you will find them. I really cannot tell you whether it is valid or not. I will say this though – the book has made it onto numerous best selling lists despite being around for many years and despite no marketing efforts. I will also say that it personally helped me to recover, although it took weeks and months of truly following the protocol described in the book.

I think it is well worth your time to examine their site and read the book in addition to following the many things I have covered in the other chapters in this book.

Flares: Some of the Worst Culprits in Causing Symptom Flare-ups

For myself, I have found certain things that tend to result in flares of my fibro symptoms. To some degree each person is different, but some of these might be more common. So, in the hope of helping my fibro-friends, here's a list of what I try to avoid that I have found to result in flares for me.

By using your daily log or mapping application, you can also isolate triggers for yourself. It is important to note these and do your best to avoid them. As I said, each person can vary considerably as to his or her symptom triggers, so you really should make your own list and work to avoid these.

Of course, there is also the factor of moderation.

Many of the items on my list might not cause a flare for me if I only indulge in small amounts, but that's just me.

Here's my list:

1. SUGAR and SIMPLE CARBS – I do best when I eliminate these completely from my diet. I replace sugar with Stevia, monk fruit, yacon syrup and coconut sugar. Depending on what I am trying to sweeten, I use different sweeteners that work best. (See other blog posts just done on alternatives to sugar).

2. ALCOHOL – I stay away from any sweet drinks, never drink on an empty stomach and never more than two drinks. When I have violated any of these points I have always been very sorry. Alcohol raises and crashes your blood sugar and often causes worsening of symptoms. A very small glass of red wine (more like half a glass) has some antioxidant benefits and can be tolerated.

3. STRESS – I can feel the cortisol pumping into my system when I am stressed. Removing all stress factors from my daily life has helped tremendously.

4. BAD SLEEP – Not getting enough sleep or a lot of disturbed sleep, particularly if over several days, can send me into a flare.

5. CAFFEINE – Caffeine initiates the production of insulin, which in turn lowers your blood sugar and leaves you with less energy. You will find that decaffeinated and herbal teas are also quite good, and once you are through some initial withdrawals, you can learn to live without coffee.

If you have to have coffee, then drink only organic decaf coffees and you really can't tell the difference.

I say organic as many coffees can have high concentrations of dangerous pesticides, so organic is important.

I use to heavily caffeinate myself to try and stay awake and I paid the price for this short and long term.

6. STAYING UP LATE – Getting good sleep has been a really important aspect of not getting flares. If I stay up late, then I often have trouble sleeping, so I have found it better to find my sweet spot of time for bed and stick to it.

7. SMOKING OR OTHER TOXINS – Smoking cigarettes or being around someone who smokes often, or if you live in or frequent an area with high levels of pollution, can result in a harmful toxic load that your body has to try and deal with. Living in an area with bad water similarly had very bad effects on my health. See more about this in another chapter.

8. TRAVELING – Whether by car or plane I usually have some backlash after a medium to longer trip.

The key is to learn what tends to trigger these flare ups and use self-discipline to avoid them. The best is a stable, steady environment with no extra stressors, no radical changes in schedule, diet, activity or stress and no toxic load on the body. However, because we don't live in an ideal world and this is not always possible, it is vital that you put in some control over your environment to avoid those factors that can knock you on your butt.

Avoiding Toxins

Keeping the toxic load in your body very low can make a big difference in how you feel.

There are many sources of toxins and damaging chemicals that can get into your body through the air you breathe, water and foods you ingest, through your skin from soaps, lotions, cosmetics, cleaning products, etc. A lot of it you just don't even realize but these toxins can build up to toxic levels in your body. Here are some of the most common ways that you can let toxins into your body

Many everyday chemicals can be a factor in the breakdown of our natural defenses against disease and overall immune system.

- Pesticides, fertilizers and other chemicals in produce
- Hormones and antibiotics found in meats, fowl and dairy

- Mercury and other heavy metals
- Preservatives and other chemicals, such as MSG in processed foods
- Many air fresheners, synthetic fragrances, aerosol sprays, perfumes, dryer sheets, laundry detergent, window cleaner and other household cleaners contain known carcinogens that can be damaging to your health.
- Air pollution, such as living near cement factory or oil refinery
- Smoking
- Cleaning products that are toxic that can absorb through your skin and that you can breathe in when you are using them. Some of these can be quite serious.
- Cooking utensils and pans made with plastic or with Teflon (or other similar type coatings) that degrade over time.
- Skin products that can be absorbed into the bloodstream through your skin that

contain carcinogens and other dangerous chemicals.

- Water that has been treated with fluoride, chlorine and other harmful chemicals.

Here's another great resource to help guide you. **http://www.ewg.org/skindeep/** has information on thousands of products including cosmetics, skin products, sunscreen, hair, nails, men's products, oral care, etc. They also have an app that you can download where you can scan any such product and it will give you the rating as to how healthy or not something is for any product in their database. Cool, huh?

www.EKG.org also has a ton of other information about foods, cleaning products and more. If you have any question about the toxic load of any products you use, check it out here. For even more information on this subject, I recommend a book entitled *Toxic Overload* by environmental health specialist Dr. Paula Baillie-Hamilton available on Amazon.

There is also a fabulous article on this by Dr. Mark Hyman which you can read here: **http://drhyman.com/blog/2010/05/19/is-there-toxic-waste-in-your-body-2/#close**

Here's what Dr. Hyman recommends that you should do:

1. ***"Drink Clean** – Drink plenty of clean water, at least eight to ten glasses of filtered water a day.*

2. ***"Eliminate Properly** – Keep your bowels moving, at least once or twice a day. And if you can't get going, then you need some help. This can include taking two tablespoons of ground flax seeds, taking acidophilus and extra magnesium citrate capsules.*

3. ***"Eat Clean** – You should also eat organic produce and animal products to eliminate the toxins, hormones, and antibiotics in your food.*

4. *"**Eat Detoxifying Food** – You should eat 8 to 10 servings of colorful fruits and vegetables a day, particularly family of the cruciferous vegetables (broccoli, collards, kale, cabbage, Brussels sprouts, kohlrabi) and the garlic family (garlic and onions), which help increase sulfur in the body and help detoxification.*

5. *"**Minimize Drugs** – Avoid stimulants, sedatives, and drugs, such as caffeine and nicotine, and try to reduce alcohol intake.*

6. *"**Get Moving** – Exercise five days a week with focus on conditioning your cardiovascular system, strengthening exercises, and stretching exercises.*

7. *"**Avoid the White Menace** – This includes white flour and white sugar.*

8. *"**Sweat** – Sweat profusely at least*

three times a week, using a sauna, steam, or a detox bath.

9. ***"Supplement*** *– Take a high-quality multivitamin and mineral supplement.*

10. ***"Relax*** *– Relax deeply every day to get your nervous system in a state of calm, rest, and relaxation."*

Tips for Traveling

Traveling can be very tricky.

I had to travel out of the country for several years and I think I ran into nearly every possible situation to be able to make a really good list of tips for traveling. So here it goes!

1. Plan ahead – book flights that don't leave too early or get you in too late, and go non-stop if at all possible. Arrive a day or two ahead of when you need to be there to allow yourself time to rest and recover from traveling before you have to be somewhere. If you are driving, then plan your travel times and stop overs so as to not do too much in a day.

2. Do your research and plan your trip well. Thoroughly check out the places you are going (your end destination as well as

any places you will stay overnight).
Check the weather thoroughly so you
know how warm or cool to dress and any
bad weather gear you may need.
Research hotels, read the reviews, search
for hotels with the best quality beds in
that area or at least the newest hotels.
Find places to eat where you can eat
healthy. Check out info about water
quality in that area as you may need to
drink only bottled water.

3.   Travel gear should be light and easy to
     handle. I never do carry-ons anymore, as
     I am always sorry about having to lug a
     bag around, particularly if you have a
     plane change. Lifting to put them into
     overhead bins is also not great either. I
     have learned to use good quality bags
     with rollers. No huge ones either, as they
     get too heavy and are unwieldy. The
     medium sized hard case bags are my

favorite. They travel well, are light, sturdy and roll easily.

4.   I do my packing over a period of many days, just a bit at a time. So as I go through the day I think of things or run across things that I should pack and I throw them into the suitcase. It is overall less stressful and I don't forget important things this way.

5.   Pack light but not too light. Research and planning is key to knowing what you are going to need for clothes, shoes, accessories, etc. You can load yourself up too much by trying to account for any possibility. Don't skimp on things you are going to need, but also be smart about shoes or jackets and jeans that can be worn with several different outfits and mix and matched to make a smaller wardrobe go a lot further. If you are

going to be in a hotel, they will have blow dryers as well as shampoo and conditioner. So cut down on what you are taking as much as possible without cutting out things you need.

6. Be as organized as possible when packing. One thing that drives me crazy is not being able to find things that I packed, so I started using luggage and smaller zippered bags that have more compartments and organization built in that make it so much easier to find the things I need.

7. Ergonomics of your travel can be very important. If you are driving or even riding in any kind of vehicle, make sure your back and neck are well supported and you are able to comfortably maintain good posture throughout the trip. If the trip is long, break it up with short or long

stopovers where you can get up, move and walk around and even rest. When we did a long road trip driving across country we paced ourselves well, took breaks throughout and stayed over a day or two in choice locations.

8. Wear comfortable shoes and clothes. Loose, comfy clothes and shoes really help. I cut out the labels from inside my clothes too. For planes I would dress warm or dress in layers as I usually get cold on a plane and am happy to have a jacket or sweater.

9. Water and food quality can vary in different states and countries. Be careful when you are in areas of lower quality or lower standards of water, produce and food preparations. Spending a day with food poisoning or drinking water with bad bacteria isn't fun. Drink bottled

water and only use higher quality restaurants. For longer trips I'd recommend staying at a place with a kitchen and buying healthy food to eat.

10. Avoid snacking on junk and eating out too much. Go to a grocery store or health food store and stock up on healthy foods that you can eat for some meals and snacks.

11. Meds, supplements and remedies: There are easier ways to pack these without having to take a million bottles. There are pill holders/organizers that you can use to put your daily vitamins/supplements and any meds in. There are even some that have compartments for morning afternoon and evening. This makes things a lot easier. Then you can use small plastic bags for any meds or supplements that are only occasional use.

This way you can still travel light and make it easy to take all of the usual things you take throughout the day.

12. Get good sleep at night and rest during the day when needed. Give yourself plenty of time to get to sleep and then sleep in late if needed. Being in different beds and different environments can affect sleep, so allow for more time to be able to get a good night's sleep. And make a point of taking short rests throughout the day when you can.

13. Exercise – get in some exercise when you can. Many hotels have elliptical machines for low impact exercise, or you can do a Canadian Air Force exercise routine or a Yoga routine in the morning before showering. Exercise produces more endorphins, which will help you to feel better throughout the day.

Producing More Endorphins

I cannot stress to you how important this is. Please don't brush it off as frivolous or unscientific.

Experiencing love and pleasure in life, whether that's from a significant other, a child or a family member, a good friend or even a pet. Or if it's your favorite pair of jeans or wildflowers in the spring, creative expression in art or music or whatever it is, it is very healthy to experience love, beauty and pleasure – and as often as possible.

Physically, your body produces endorphins when you experience pleasure, when you smile (a real smile, not a fake one), when you laugh, and when you feel love. Your body also produces endorphins when you exercise. These endorphins are chemicals in your brain that improve your mood, decrease stress, enhance pleasure and also help the body to heal.

So, really, it is very, very important to your own healing to experience beauty, pleasure and love as much as possible.

I am incredibly fortunate to have a husband who has been an angel-extraordinaire. He has taken such good care of me and has seen me through some very dark times. I am eternally grateful to him for so many things that it would take an entire book to list them. We have a strong and powerful love. And it is that love that I must acknowledge as an integral part of my healing.

Love, whether from a spouse, another family member, a dear friend or a loving pet, is a vital part of any treatment plan.

Don't under-estimate the power of love in your road to recovery.

Checklist of Things that Help

I am going to lay out here a short summary of what I have found to be most beneficial and helpful.

This is something you can review often, and as you have tried each yourself - either newly or in the past – you can mark those points that you have found to be helpful for you. You can also add others factors that you have found by other means that are not on this list and end up with a tailored list for you of all the things that improve your condition.

You can also review your journal to analyze good and bad days and anything noted that contributed to improvement or worsening. This may give you additional points you want to add to the list.

What has helped me and I classified as valid and useful treatments:

—Getting good sleep – there are many supplements and handlings you can do to get good sleep each night, and the ones I know are covered in this book and on my website.

—Handling any nutritional deficiencies with healthy diet and supplements including vitamin D, minerals and trace minerals, omega 3 oil, and protein.

—Handling any infections – whether bacterial, viral, yeast or other infestations – under a doctor's care.

—Handling any hormonal deficiencies with bio-identical hormone therapy under the care and direction of a competent doctor.

—Exercise: Probably the most important of all. It is important that such exercise includes a proper warm-up, stretching, cardio and muscle strengthening. Make sure to go very, very light and build up very gradually. Do not overdo it. The Royal Canadian Air Force exercises, Yoga, swimming and water exercises are all good choices, but certainly are not the only options.

—Heat and particularly wet heat. This could be a long, hot shower, a hot bath with Epsom Salts, an infrared sauna or heat-packs.

—Getting rid of or greatly lessening the stress in every aspect of your life – work, home, relationships, financial, etc.

—Healthy eating: Some of this is outlined here in this book, but much more is covered in another book I am writing called *HealthKick: Easy Healthy Living Hacks* – which you will find on Amazon Kindle.

—Drinking a lot of fluids, preferably water, and keeping yourself well hydrated.

—Cut out the caffeine, nicotine, sugar and simple carbs. These are your enemies. Instead eat lots of vegetables, lean proteins and balanced meals.

—Avoid toxins as much as possible, such as many cleaning products, pesticides, hair and skin products, air pollution, tap water in some areas, smoking, etc.

—Avoid taking prescription pain or anti-depressant drugs if at all possible or work to phase them out as you can. The long-term use of OTC pain meds can also have bad side effects so these also should only be used when absolutely necessary and phased out as soon as possible.

—Good posture, good work and sleep ergonomics. Specifically, I recommend the Gokhale method.

—Proper breathing techniques.

—Physical therapy and massage, which includes the common trigger points.

—Chiropractic adjustments, as long as they are gentle and also use heat and massage.

—Comfortable shoes and clothes.

—A good mattress that has a thin layer of soft cushion but also has excellent support.

—Guaifenesin regimen – if also accompanied by not using skin products with salicylates.

—Avoiding common or known triggers.

—Be happy – do things you love and enjoy as much as you can. Cherish and be grateful for the good things in your life.

Spend time with those you love and do all you can to experience happiness. Healing the soul can go a long way toward healing the body.

Conclusion

Thank you so very much for taking the time to read my book. If I can impart information that helps to relieve any of your symptoms, I will consider that my work has been of some value.

I have tried to make this as to the point and as informative as possible. I also have a website with more information and tools. It is **www.FibromyalgiaFree.org**. Please feel free to contact me directly through that website so that I can answer any other questions you have or be of any assistance to you.

If you got anything helpful from this book, then I would be incredibly grateful and forever thankful if you would write a review of the book on Amazon. This will help me reach more people that are afflicted with chronic illness that can be helped. Thank you in advance for taking the time out to do this. It really does help a lot and is deeply appreciated.

Fibro-free is a division of HealthKick, which covers a broader range of Health topics.

You can find out more about HealthKick at **http://www.HealthKick.info/** and you can subscribe to our blog by hitting the orange subscribe button on the right side.

You can also connect with me through my social media:

Facebook:
https://www.facebook.com/debbiebaumgarten

Twitter:
twitter.com/healthkickguru

Pinterest:
www.pinterest.com/debbiebaumgarte/

LinkedIn:
www.linkedin.com/profile/view?id=337802198

I would love to hear from you and I will do my best to always answer promptly.

Write me and ask me questions. I am so happy to help anyone I can in any way I can. Thank you again for taking the time to consider what I have laid out here. You are in my thoughts and in my heart. I sincerely hope you heal and get better.

ABOUT THE AUTHOR

Debbie was diagnosed with Fibromyalgia in 2000 at the Mayo Clinic. This was following many years of self-abuse – smoking, excessive caffeine, poor and erratic sleep, combined with lots of stress. The pain and debilitating fatigue became completely overwhelming.

Debbie embarked on extensive research, study and visits to clinics to better understand her condition and to recover her health.

After years of trials, she mapped her own way to a recovery of her health.

Debbie has written her books to make it as easy as possible for others to understand what is most important about healthy living and to help those suffering with chronic illness.

Accomplishing this through her books for thousands of people is her dream.

Debbie founded Fibro-Free which you can visit at **www.FibromyalgiaFree.org** to provide helpful information to those suffering from Fibromyalgia, Chronic Fatigue or Chronic

Illness as a means of relaying the best and most important information and treatments for recovery from these debilitating syndromes and diseases.

She founded HealthKick as a means of simplifying healthy living information and making it as easy as possible to eat and live using healthier habits. She wrote her second book, *HealthKick, Easy Healthy Living Hacks,* to accomplish this. This will be available on Amazon Kindle. The HealthKick website and blog – **http://www.HealthKick.info** – is also packed full of information, with more added almost everyday.

Her next book, *Is Sugar Killing Me? The Healthy Alternatives*, focuses more on the dangers of sugar consumption as a leading cause of obesity and thus obesity related diseases and disabilities.

Here she investigates alternatives to sugar, exposing the dangers of artificial sweeteners and explaining the best options in natural sweeteners that can be used as alternatives to sugar.

Based on her research, she founded Sin Free Desserts – www.sinfreedesserts.com – introducing a line of desserts that are: free of sugar, free of any artificial sweeteners, wheat and gluten free, additives and preservatives free, low in carbs, high in protein, high in fiber and that contain good omega 3 oils. In other words, she has discovered ways to indulge that are actually good for you.

While her loves are her husband and living in the Texas Hill Country, her passion is helping others live healthy, pain-free and happy lives.